SOMATIC YOGA EXERCISES

45 Mind Body Exercises To Reduce Stress, Relieve Anxiety And Lose Weight Quickly With 60 Day Challenge

DR. PERSIS HILLARY

Copyright 2024

This book is a copyrighted work, and all rights are reserved by the author. No part of this publication may be reproduced, distributed, or transmitted in any form or by any means, including photocopying, recording, or other electronic or mechanical methods, without the prior written permission of the author, except in the case of brief quotations embodied in critical reviews and certain other noncommercial uses permitted by copyright law.

TABLE OF CONTENTS

WHAT IS SOMATIC YOGA EXERCISE

Somatic Yoga Exercise is an intriguing and unique approach to yoga that combines traditional yoga practices with somatic exercises. It's essential to understand that "somatic" refers to the body in its wholeness, particularly as perceived from within. This concept is central to understanding the purpose and methodology of Somatic Yoga.

Origin and Philosophy

Somatic Yoga is rooted in the principles of somatics, a field of study and practice that emphasizes internal physical perception and experience. The term "somatic" is derived from the Greek word "soma," meaning the living body in its entirety – muscles, tissues, senses, and emotions. This approach contrasts with traditional views of the body as merely a mechanical structure.

Core Principles

1. Mind-Body Integration: It focuses on the mind-body connection, emphasizing awareness of the body's internal state. This heightened awareness is believed to promote a deeper understanding and control over one's physical and mental well-being.

2. Gentle Movements: Somatic Yoga involves gentle, mindful movements that are aimed at re-educating the body. These movements are designed to release tension, improve flexibility, and enhance bodily control.

3. Self-Perception and Awareness: A significant aspect of Somatic Yoga is developing a heightened sense of self-perception and awareness. Practitioners are encouraged to pay close attention to their bodily sensations and responses during exercises.

Techniques and Practices

- Somatic Movements: These are slow, gentle, and often repetitive movements that help to increase body awareness and release muscle tension.

- Breathwork: Breathing techniques are a critical part of Somatic Yoga, used to deepen relaxation and increase body awareness.

- Mindfulness and Meditation: Integral to Somatic Yoga, these practices foster a deep connection between the mind and the body.

- Yoga Postures: Traditional yoga postures are integrated but performed with a greater focus on internal sensations and mindfulness.

Benefits

- Stress Reduction: The mindful and introspective nature of Somatic Yoga can lead to significant stress reduction.

- Improved Flexibility and Mobility: By focusing on internal sensations and gentle movements, it can improve flexibility and joint mobility.

- Body Awareness: Practitioners often report an increased awareness of their bodies, leading to better posture and movement in daily life.

- Pain Management: Somatic Yoga has been found helpful in managing chronic pain, particularly pain related to muscular tension and misalignment.

Somatic Yoga Exercise offers a unique blend of yoga and somatic practices, emphasizing internal body awareness and mindful movement. It's particularly beneficial for those looking to deepen their mind-body connection, reduce stress, and improve physical mobility. By focusing on gentle, introspective practices, it provides a path to better understand and care for one's body and mind.

HOW TO USE THIS GUIDE EFFECTIVELY

To use a guide on somatic yoga exercises effectively, follow these steps:

1. Understand Somatic Yoga: Before you start, ensure you have a basic understanding of what somatic yoga is. It's a form of yoga that focuses on internal physical perception and experience. The aim is to enhance mind-body integration through physical movements.

2. Read Through the Guide: Go through the entire guide first to get an overview of the exercises, their purposes, and any special instructions or precautions.

3. Set Realistic Goals: Determine what you want to achieve with somatic yoga. It could be increased flexibility, stress reduction, better body awareness, or improved posture.

4. Create a Routine: Based on the guide, create a yoga routine that fits into your daily schedule. Consistency is key in yoga practice.

5. Prepare Your Space: Ensure you have a comfortable, quiet space to practice. Use a yoga mat or a soft surface to perform the exercises.

6. Practice Mindfulness: Somatic yoga emphasizes internal awareness. Pay close attention to your body's sensations, emotions, and thoughts as you perform each exercise.

7. Go at Your Own Pace: Don't rush the movements. Somatic yoga is about exploring and understanding your body, not pushing it to its limits.

8. Use the Guide as a Reference: During your practice, refer back to the guide for proper techniques, breathing patterns, and alignment tips.

9. Incorporate Breathing Exercises: Somatic yoga often involves specific breathing techniques. Make sure you understand and apply these as instructed in the guide.

10. Listen to Your Body: If any exercise causes pain or discomfort, stop immediately. Somatic yoga is about gentle exploration and should not cause pain.

11. Track Your Progress: Keep a journal of your practice, noting how different exercises affect your body and mind. This can help you tailor your practice to your needs.

12. Seek Professional Advice if Needed: If you have any health concerns or if you're new to yoga, consult a healthcare provider or a qualified yoga instructor.

Remember, the effectiveness of somatic yoga, like any other yoga practice, largely depends on your commitment, consistency, and mindfulness during practice.

EXERCISES

1. Arch and Flatten

This exercise involves movements to enhance spinal flexibility and core engagement.

- Starting Position: Lie on your back on a comfortable, flat surface. Keep your knees bent with your feet flat on the ground, hip-width apart.

- Execution:

  - Arch: Inhale deeply. Gently tilt your pelvis backward, creating an arch in your lower back. You'll feel a slight gap between your back and the floor.

  - Flatten: Exhale slowly. Now, tilt your pelvis forward, pressing your lower back into the floor. Engage your abdominal muscles during this motion.

  - Repeat: Continue alternating between arching and flattening your back, synchronizing the movements with your breath.

2. Cat-Cow Stretch

This yoga-based exercise enhances spinal flexibility and soothes tension in the back and neck.

- Starting Position: Get on your hands and knees in a tabletop position. Ensure your knees are under your hips and your wrists under your shoulders.

- Execution:

  - Cat: Exhale and round your spine towards the ceiling, tucking your chin to your chest, creating a shape like a Halloween cat.

  - Cow: Inhale and lift your head and tailbone towards the sky, allowing your belly to sink towards the floor.

  - Repeat: Alternate between the Cat and Cow positions, flowing smoothly from one to the other.

3. Pelvic Clock

This exercise is aimed at increasing awareness and control of the pelvic movements.

- Starting Position: Lie on your back with your knees bent and feet flat on the floor. Imagine a clock laid flat on your pelvis, with 12 o'clock towards your head and 6 o'clock towards your feet.

- Execution:

  - Gently tilt your pelvis towards each 'hour' on the clock in a smooth, controlled manner. For instance, tilting towards 12 o'clock then 6 o'clock, and side to side from 3 to 9 o'clock.

  - Explore diagonal movements, like moving between 1 and 7 o'clock, then 11 and 5 o'clock.

  - The movement should be subtle and controlled.

4. Diagonal Arch and Curl

This exercise integrates torso movements to enhance coordination and core strength.

- Starting Position: Lie on your back with your knees bent and feet flat on the ground.

- Execution:

  - Lift one arm overhead while extending the opposite leg, creating a diagonal stretch.

  - Return to the starting position and switch sides, lifting the other arm and the opposite leg.

  - Focus on smooth, controlled movements, keeping your core engaged.

5. Hip Rolling

A great exercise for hip mobility and lower back relaxation.

- Starting Position: Lie on your back with your knees bent and feet flat on the ground, hip-width apart.

- Execution:

  - Keep your feet together and knees bent. Gently roll your knees to one side, allowing your hips to follow, but keep your shoulders on the ground.

  - Return to the center and then roll to the other side.

- Move in a controlled manner, feeling the rotation through your lower spine and hips.

6. Hamstring Pandiculation

Pandiculation is a technique often used in somatic exercises to help release tension and lengthen muscles.

1. Starting Position: Stand upright, feet shoulder-width apart.

2. Bend Forward: Slowly bend forward at the hips, keeping your back straight. Reach towards your toes.

3. Contract Hamstrings: While in the bent position, gently contract your hamstrings for a few seconds. You should feel a gentle pull but no discomfort.

4. Release and Stretch: Slowly release the hamstring contraction and try to stretch a little further towards your toes.

5. Return to Standing: Gradually return to the standing position.

6. Repeat: Do this a few times, each time trying to increase the stretch gently.

7. Shoulder Lift and Drop

This exercise helps to relieve tension in the shoulders and neck.

1. Starting Position: Stand or sit comfortably with your arms at your sides.

2. Lift Shoulders: Inhale and lift your shoulders towards your ears as high as you can.

3. Hold and Tense: Hold this position for a few seconds, tensing the shoulder muscles.

4. Drop Shoulders: Exhale and let your shoulders drop back down.

5. Repeat: Do this several times, feeling the tension release with each drop.

8. Neck Slow Rolls

This exercise promotes flexibility and relief in the neck area.

1. Starting Position: Sit or stand upright.

2. Chin to Chest: Gently lower your chin towards your chest.

3. Side Roll: Slowly roll your head towards one shoulder, then back down to your chest, and over to the other shoulder in a smooth motion.

4. Backward Roll: If comfortable, continue the roll slightly backward but be careful not to strain your neck.

5. Repeat: Perform this slowly, feeling the stretch in different parts of your neck. Do it in both directions.

9. Side Bend Stretch

The side bend stretch targets the muscles of the sides, improving flexibility.

1. Starting Position: Stand with feet shoulder-width apart.

2. Lateral Bend: Raise one arm overhead and bend your torso to the opposite side. Keep your other arm down by your side.

3. Hold the Stretch: Hold the stretch for a few seconds, feeling it along the side of your body.

4. Return to Center: Slowly come back to the starting position.

5. Switch Sides: Repeat the same on the other side.

10. Spinal Rotation

This exercise is excellent for lower back flexibility and spinal health.

1. Starting Position: Sit on a chair or on the floor with legs crossed.

2. Rotate Torso: Turn your upper body to one side, placing your hand on the opposite knee for a gentle twist. The other hand can rest behind you for support.

3. Hold the Position: Hold this position for a few seconds, breathing normally.

4. Return to Center: Slowly return to the center.

5. Repeat on Opposite Side: Do the same on the other side.

11. Cobra Pose Pandiculation

Cobra Pose Pandiculation is a variant of the traditional Cobra Pose, integrated with the concept of pandiculation, which involves a conscious, controlled stretch and contraction of muscles.

- Starting Position: Lie face down on a mat, legs extended, feet hip-width apart, and the tops of your feet resting on the mat.

- Hand Placement: Place your hands under your shoulders, palms down.

- Initial Movement: Gently press your hands into the mat, slowly lifting your head, shoulders, and chest off the ground. Keep your elbows close to your body.

- Pandiculation: As you lift into the Cobra Pose, begin a deep, deliberate stretch from the lower back through the spine to the neck. Then, intentionally contract the muscles along the spine.

- Hold and Release: Hold this position for a few seconds, consciously feeling the stretch and contraction. Then, slowly lower back down to the starting position.

12. Somatic Child's Pose

Somatic Child's Pose focuses on a mindful, body-awareness approach to the traditional Child's Pose.

- Starting Position: Kneel on a mat with your big toes touching and knees apart.

- Movement: Sit back on your heels and fold forward, extending your arms in front of you with palms on the mat.

- Somatic Focus: As you hold the pose, pay attention to the sensations in your hips, back, and shoulders. Breathe deeply and allow any tension to release with each exhalation.

- Duration: Stay in this position for several breaths, focusing on the sensations and relaxing more deeply into the pose with each breath.

13. Somatic Downward Dog

In Somatic Downward Dog, the emphasis is on internal bodily sensations and mindfulness, rather than perfect form.

- Starting Position: Begin in a tabletop position - hands under shoulders, knees under hips.

- Transition: Lift your hips upwards, straightening your legs and arms, forming an inverted V shape.

- Somatic Awareness: Pay attention to how your body feels in this position. Notice areas of tightness or ease. Adjust the pose to what feels right for your body, rather than striving for a textbook pose.

- Breathing: Breathe deeply, and with each exhale, try to release tension in the body.

14. Steeple Twist

Steeple Twist is a seated, spinal twist exercise that promotes flexibility and spinal health.

- Starting Position: Sit on a mat with your legs extended in front of you.

- Leg Movement: Bend your right knee and place your right foot flat on the floor outside your left knee.

- Upper Body Twist: Place your left elbow outside your right knee and your right hand on the floor behind you for support.

- Twisting Action: Gently twist your torso to the right, looking over your right shoulder. Keep your spine elongated.

- Hold and Switch Sides: Hold this twist for several breaths, then release and repeat on the other side.

15. Walking Warrior Pose

Walking Warrior Pose is a dynamic version of the Warrior Pose, adding movement to the traditional static pose.

- Starting Position: Stand tall with feet together.

- Step and Lower: Step your right foot forward into a lunge, bending your right knee at a 90-degree angle. Raise your arms overhead, palms facing each other.

- Movement: Push off with your left foot, bringing it forward next to your right as you lower your arms.

- Repeat: Step forward with your left foot, entering the lunge on the other side. Continue this walking motion, alternating sides.

Absolutely! Let's go through each of these exercises step-by-step, explaining them in a clear and unique way.

16. Somatic Bridge

The Somatic Bridge exercise is a variation of the traditional bridge pose, focusing on mindful movements and body awareness.

1. Starting Position: Lie on your back on a comfortable surface, with your knees bent and feet flat on the ground, hip-width apart. Keep your arms at your sides, palms facing down.

2. Initial Lift: Slowly lift your hips towards the ceiling, focusing on engaging your glutes and hamstrings. Keep your feet and shoulders firmly planted on the ground.

3. Mindful Movement: As you lift, pay attention to how your body feels. Notice the stretching of the hip flexors and the engagement of the lower back.

4. Peak and Hold: Once you've reached a comfortable height, hold the position for a few breaths, maintaining a conscious connection with the muscles being used.

5. Slow Descent: Carefully lower your hips back to the starting position, vertebra by vertebra, staying aware of the movement.

17. Hip Flexor Release

This exercise aims to relieve tension in the hip flexors, which is essential for those who sit for long periods.

1. Starting Position: Stand upright, then take a large step forward with one foot, keeping the other foot behind you.

2. Lower into Lunge: Bend your front knee to lower into a lunge position. Your back leg should be straight, with the heel lifted off the ground.

3. Hip Forward: Gently push your hips forward, keeping your upper body straight. You should feel a stretch in the front of your hip on the back leg.

4. Hold and Breathe: Hold this position for about 30 seconds, breathing deeply and focusing on the stretch in the hip flexor.

5. Switch Sides: Return to the starting position and repeat the exercise with the other leg.

18. Somatic Pigeon Pose

This variation of the pigeon pose emphasizes internal awareness and relaxation of the muscles.

1. Starting Position: Begin on all fours in a tabletop position.

2. Knee Forward: Bring one knee forward, placing it behind your wrist while angling the foot towards the opposite hip.

3. Extend Back Leg: Stretch your back leg straight behind you, keeping your hips square to the ground.

4. Lower Down: Slowly lower your torso down, either staying on your hands or coming down to your forearms or chest for a deeper stretch.

5. Mindful Engagement: Focus on the sensations in your hip and glute of the bent leg, breathing deeply and allowing any tension to release.

6. Hold and Switch: Maintain the pose for up to a minute, then slowly come out and switch to the other leg.

19. Standing Side Stretch

A simple but effective stretch for the sides of the body, improving flexibility and relieving tension.

1. Starting Position: Stand with your feet together and arms by your sides.

2. Raise Arms: Lift your arms overhead, clasping your fingers together.

3. Lean to Side: Gently lean to one side, keeping your arms straight and stretching the opposite side of your body.

4. Hold and Breathe: Hold the stretch for about 20-30 seconds, breathing deeply and feeling the stretch along your side.

5. Repeat Other Side: Return to the starting position and repeat the stretch on the other side.

20. Somatic Tree Pose

A mindful variation of the tree pose that enhances balance and focuses on bodily sensations.

1. Starting Position: Stand straight with your feet hip-width apart.

2. Foot to Thigh: Shift your weight to one foot and place the sole of the other foot on the inner thigh or calf (avoid the knee) of the standing leg.

3. Balance and Align: Bring your hands together in front of your chest in a prayer position, focusing on a fixed point for balance.

4. Mindful Awareness: As you balance, be aware of your body's micro-adjustments to maintain the pose. Feel the groundedness of your standing foot and the engagement of your core.

5. Hold and Switch: Maintain the pose for 30 seconds to a minute, then gently lower your foot and switch sides.

21. Gentle Backbend:

- Start by lying on your back on a comfortable surface, with your knees bent and feet flat on the ground.

- Place your arms alongside your body, palms facing down.

- Gradually lift your pelvis and lower back off the ground by pushing through your feet, engaging your glutes and lower back muscles.

- Keep your shoulders and head relaxed on the ground.

- Hold the lift for a few seconds, feeling a gentle stretch in your chest and abdomen.

- Gently lower your back to the starting position.

- This exercise helps to stretch the front of the body and strengthen the back muscles.

22. Somatic Forward Bend:

- Stand with your feet hip-width apart, knees slightly bent.

- Inhale deeply, and as you exhale, slowly bend forward from your hips, not the waist.

- Let your head and arms hang loosely towards the ground.

- Focus on the sensations in your body, noticing any areas of tension or relaxation.

- Breathe deeply and gently sway side to side if comfortable.

- To rise, roll up slowly, one vertebra at a time, keeping your head to come up last.

- This exercise helps in releasing tension in the back and enhancing body awareness.

23. Butterfly Pose with Somatic Awareness:

- Sit on the floor with a straight spine.

- Bring the soles of your feet together, allowing your knees to fall out to the sides.

- Hold your feet with your hands, and gently flap your knees up and down like the wings of a butterfly.

- Focus on the sensations in your hips and inner thighs.

- Optionally, lean forward to intensify the stretch, keeping your back straight.

- Breathe deeply and maintain the pose for a few minutes.

- This pose helps in opening the hips and improving flexibility.

24. Side-Lying Leg Lifts:

- Lie on your side with your legs extended, one on top of the other.

- Rest your head on your lower arm or a pillow for support.

- Keeping your top leg straight, lift it upwards, engaging the muscles in your outer thigh and hip.

- Slowly lower it back down.

- Perform several repetitions before switching to the other side.

- This exercise strengthens the muscles on the sides of your hips and thighs.

25. Somatic Plank:

- Begin in a face-down position on the floor, with your elbows under your shoulders, forearms on the ground.

- Lift your body so that it forms a straight line from your head to your heels.

- Engage your core muscles, and be mindful of the sensations throughout your body.

- Keep your gaze down and neck neutral.

- Hold this position for several seconds, breathing evenly.

- Lower your body back to the starting position.

- This version of the plank focuses on body awareness and core strength.

26. Somatic Triangle Pose

1. Starting Position: Stand with your feet wide apart, around 3-4 feet. Turn your right foot out 90 degrees and your left foot in slightly.

2. Arms: Extend your arms to the sides at shoulder height, palms facing down.

3. Movement: Shift your hips to the left, and then extend your torso to the right, directly over the right leg.

4. Hand Placement: Lower your right hand towards your ankle, shin, or the floor outside your right foot. Your left arm should stretch upwards towards the ceiling, fingers pointing up. Ensure both arms form a straight line.

5. Gaze and Hold: Turn your gaze to look at your left hand. Hold this pose while breathing deeply for 30-60 seconds.

6. Return and Repeat: To release, inhale and press your feet firmly into the floor, reaching your left arm upwards to come back up. Turn your feet forward and lower your arms. Repeat on the other side.

27. Knee-to-Chest Release

1. Starting Position: Lie on your back with your legs extended and arms at your sides.

2. Movement: Bend your right knee and bring it towards your chest.

3. Grip: Interlace your fingers just below the knee or on the shin, but avoid placing them directly on the knee cap.

4. Hold: Gently pull the knee closer to the chest, feeling a stretch in the lower back and hip. Hold for 20-30 seconds, breathing deeply.

5. Release and Repeat: Slowly release the right leg back to the starting position and repeat the same on the left leg.

28. Somatic Warrior II

1. Starting Position: Stand with your feet wide apart, about 3-4 feet. Turn your right foot out 90 degrees and your left foot in slightly.

2. Arm Position: Extend your arms to the sides at shoulder height, palms facing down.

3. Bend Right Knee: Bend your right knee so it's over your right ankle, thigh parallel to the floor. Your left leg should be straight.

4. Gaze and Hold: Turn your head to look over your right hand. Hold this position, breathing deeply for about 30-60 seconds.

5. Return and Repeat: To release, straighten your right knee, lower your arms, and turn your feet forward. Repeat on the left side.

29. Ankle Circles

1. Starting Position: Sit or lie down in a comfortable position. Extend one leg.

2. Movement: Lift the extended leg slightly and start rotating the ankle. Make 10-15 circles in a clockwise direction.

3. Reverse Direction: Now rotate the same ankle counterclockwise for 10-15 circles.

4. Switch Legs: Lower the leg and repeat the same process with the other ankle.

30. Somatic Squat

1. Starting Position: Stand with your feet slightly wider than shoulder-width apart, toes pointing forward.

2. Arm Position: Extend your arms straight out in front of you for balance.

3. Squat Down: Bend your knees and lower your hips as if you are sitting back in a chair. Keep your back straight and chest lifted.

4. Depth and Hold: Go as low as you can without compromising your form. Your knees should not go past your toes. Hold at the lowest point for a few seconds.

5. Rise Up: Push through your heels to return to the starting position.

31. Somatic Eagle Pose

1. Starting Position: Stand with your feet hip-width apart.

2. Arms: Stretch your arms forward, parallel to the floor. Cross your right arm over the left, bend your elbows, and try to bring your palms together. If that's difficult, touch the backs of your hands together or grab your opposite shoulder.

3. Legs: Bend your knees slightly. Lift your right foot, cross it over your left thigh, and if possible, hook your right foot behind your left calf.

4. Balance and Hold: Focus on balancing while you breathe deeply. Imagine the sensation of energy flowing through your intertwined limbs.

5. Release and Repeat: Unwind your arms and legs, then repeat on the opposite side.

32. Cross-Legged Twist

1. Starting Position: Sit on the floor with your legs crossed.

2. Twist Setup: Place your right hand behind you for support. Bring your left hand to your right knee.

3. Execute the Twist: Inhale deeply, lengthening your spine. As you exhale, gently twist to the right. Lead the movement from your abdomen, allowing your gaze to follow naturally.

4. Maintain and Breathe: Hold the twist for a few breaths, focusing on the sensation of your muscles contracting and releasing.

5. Release and Repeat: Slowly return to the center and repeat the twist on the opposite side.

33. Somatic Crescent Lunge

1. Starting Position: Stand and step your right foot back into a lunge, keeping your left knee over your ankle.

2. Arm Position: Raise your arms overhead, palms facing each other.

3. Lunge Deepening: Sink deeper into the lunge, focusing on the stretch in your right hip flexor and the strength in your left thigh.

4. Breathing and Awareness: Breathe deeply, bringing awareness to the sensations in your hips and spine.

5. Return and Switch: Return to standing and switch sides, stepping your left foot back.

34. Somatic Goddess Pose

1. Starting Position: Stand with your feet wider than hip-width apart, toes pointing out.

2. Lowering into the Pose: Bend your knees, lowering into a squat. Aim to get your thighs parallel to the ground.

3. Arm Position: Bring your arms to a 'cactus' position, elbows bent at 90 degrees, palms facing forward.

4. Engage and Breathe: Engage your core and glutes. Breathe deeply, feeling the openness in your hips and chest.

5. Maintain and Release: Hold for several breaths, then straighten your legs to release.

35. Somatic Half Moon Pose

1. Starting Position: Begin in a standing forward fold.

2. Transition: Place your right hand on the ground (or a block) about a foot in front of your right foot, slightly to the right side.

3. Lifting into Pose: Shift your weight onto your right foot and lift your left leg up, aligning it with your torso.

4. Arm Position: Extend your left arm towards the ceiling, opening your chest.

5. Alignment and Focus: Keep your gaze focused on a point for balance. Feel the stretch and alignment from your left fingertips through your left foot.

6. Hold and Switch Sides: Maintain the pose for a few breaths, then gently come out and repeat on the other side.

36. Somatic Chair Pose

This exercise is a variation of the traditional Chair Pose in yoga, but with a focus on somatic awareness, which means being acutely aware of your body's sensations and movements.

1. Starting Position: Stand with your feet hip-width apart. Engage your core and keep your back straight.

2. Entering the Pose: As you inhale, raise your arms overhead, keeping them parallel. Exhale and bend your knees, pushing your hips back as if you are about to sit in a chair.

3. Alignment Focus: Ensure your knees don't go beyond your toes. Distribute your weight evenly on your feet.

4. Somatic Awareness: Pay attention to the sensations in your thighs, calves, and back. Notice the stretching and contracting of muscles.

5. Duration: Hold the pose for 5-10 breaths, focusing on the sensations in your body.

6. Exiting the Pose: Inhale and straighten your legs, lowering your arms.

37. Somatic Mountain Pose

This is a mindful version of the Mountain Pose, emphasizing body awareness.

1. Starting Position: Stand with your feet together, arms by your side.

2. Engaging the Body: Engage your thigh muscles slightly, drawing up your kneecaps. Tuck your tailbone slightly, but keep the natural curve of your back.

3. Arm and Shoulder Alignment: Let your arms hang naturally with palms facing forward. Relax your shoulders down and back.

4. Somatic Focus: Close your eyes and focus on the sensations in your feet, legs, and spine. Feel the grounding of your feet and the lift of your spine.

5. Breathing: Breathe deeply and steadily, maintaining the pose for at least 30 seconds.

6. Exiting the Pose: Relax your muscles and then step out of the pose.

38. Shoulder Blade Squeeze

This exercise helps in improving posture and strengthening the muscles around the shoulder blades.

1. Starting Position: Stand or sit with your back straight.

2. Movement: Pull your shoulder blades towards each other, as if trying to hold a pencil between them.

3. Alignment: Keep your neck long and shoulders away from your ears.

4. Somatic Awareness: Notice the contraction between your shoulder blades and the release of tension in your shoulders.

5. Hold and Release: Hold the squeeze for 5 seconds and then gently release. Repeat 8-10 times.

39. Somatic Fish Pose

A variation of the Fish Pose with a focus on internal sensations.

1. Starting Position: Lie on your back with your legs extended and arms by your side.

2. Entering the Pose: Press your forearms and elbows into the floor and lift your chest to create an arch in your upper back.

3. Head Position: Let your head tilt back gently, opening your throat. Ensure not to strain your neck.

4. Somatic Awareness: Focus on the stretching sensation in your chest and throat.

5. Breathing: Maintain deep, steady breaths. Hold for 15-30 seconds.

6. Exiting the Pose: Lower your back and head gently to the floor.

40. Somatic Bow Pose

This is a mindful approach to the Bow Pose, focusing on the body's internal experience.

1. Starting Position: Lie on your stomach with your hands by your sides.

2. Preparation: Bend your knees and reach back to grab the outside of your ankles.

3. Lifting into the Pose: As you inhale, lift your heels away from your buttocks and simultaneously lift your head and chest off the floor.

4. Alignment and Focus: Keep your knees hip-width apart. Focus on the stretch in your shoulders, chest, thighs, and abdomen.

5. Breathing: Breathe deeply, maintaining the pose for 20-30 seconds.

6. Releasing the Pose: Exhale, gently release your legs and lower your chest to the floor.

41. Wrist Flexion and Extension:

- Step 1: Begin by sitting or standing with your back straight and shoulders relaxed.

- Step 2: Extend your arms in front of you at shoulder height.

- Step 3: Keep your palms facing down and fingers pointing forward.

- Step 4: Slowly flex your wrists by moving your fingers towards the floor. You should feel a gentle stretch in your forearms.

- Step 5: Hold the flexed position for 15-30 seconds while maintaining slow, controlled breathing.

- Step 6: Return to the starting position with your palms facing down.

- Step 7: Now, extend your wrists by moving your fingers towards the ceiling. Feel the stretch in your wrists and forearms.

- Step 8: Hold the extended position for 15-30 seconds, continuing to breathe deeply.

- Step 9: Repeat the flexion and extension movements for 2-3 sets, gradually increasing the duration of the stretch as you become more comfortable.

42. Somatic Camel Pose:

- Step 1: Begin by kneeling on the floor with your knees hip-width apart.

- Step 2: Place your hands on your lower back, fingers pointing downward.

- Step 3: Inhale deeply, arch your back, and gently push your hips forward.

- Step 4: As you arch your back, tilt your head back and look up towards the ceiling.

- Step 5: Hold this pose for 15-30 seconds while breathing deeply and maintaining balance.

- Step 6: Exhale and slowly return to the kneeling position.

- Step 7: Repeat the camel pose 2-3 times, gradually increasing the duration of the stretch.

43. Somatic Revolved Triangle:

- Step 1: Begin in a standing position with your feet about hip-width apart.

- Step 2: Extend your arms out to the sides at shoulder height.

- Step 3: Pivot your left foot 90 degrees to the left and your right foot slightly to the left.

- Step 4: Inhale deeply, then exhale and reach your left hand towards your right foot, bending at the waist.

- Step 5: Place your left hand on the outside of your right foot, or on a block if flexibility is limited.

- Step 6: Extend your right arm upwards towards the ceiling, opening your chest.

- Step 7: Hold this twisted triangle pose for 15-30 seconds while breathing deeply.

- Step 8: Inhale and return to the starting position.

- Step 9: Repeat on the other side by pivoting your right foot and reaching with your right hand.

44. Somatic Dancer's Pose:

- Step 1: Begin by standing tall with your feet hip-width apart.

- Step 2: Shift your weight to your left leg and bend your right knee.

- Step 3: Reach your right hand behind you and hold your right ankle.

- Step 4: Extend your left arm straight out in front of you for balance.

- Step 5: Inhale deeply and begin to lift your right foot towards the ceiling, simultaneously arching your back.

- Step 6: Hold the dancer's pose for 15-30 seconds while maintaining your balance and breathing deeply.

- Step 7: Slowly release your right ankle and return to a standing position.

- Step 8: Repeat on the other side by shifting your weight to your right leg and bending your left knee.

45. Pelvic Tilts in Supine Position:

- Step 1: Lie on your back with your knees bent and feet flat on the floor.

- Step 2: Place your arms by your sides with your palms facing down.

- Step 3: Inhale deeply, then exhale and engage your core muscles.

- Step 4: Tilt your pelvis upward by pressing your lower back into the floor. Your tailbone should lift slightly.

- Step 5: Hold this pelvic tilt for a few seconds while continuing to breathe.

- Step 6: Inhale and release the tilt, allowing your lower back to gently arch away from the floor.

- Step 7: Exhale and repeat the pelvic tilt 10-15 times, focusing on the movement of your pelvis.

TIPS FOR STAYING ON THE SOAMTIC YOGA EXERCISE

1. Start with Breath Awareness: Begin each session by focusing on your breath. Pay attention to the natural rhythm of your breath.

2. Create a Quiet Space: Find a quiet and peaceful environment for your practice to minimize distractions.

3. Use a Yoga Mat: Practice on a yoga mat or comfortable surface to provide cushioning and stability.

4. Wear Comfortable Clothing: Choose loose-fitting, comfortable clothing that allows for easy movement.

5. Set an Intention: Set a positive intention or affirmation for your practice to create a sense of purpose.

6. Warm-Up Gradually: Start with gentle warm-up movements to prepare your body for deeper stretches.

7. Move Mindfully: Practice each movement slowly and mindfully, focusing on the sensations in your body.

8. Stay Present: Keep your attention on the present moment, letting go of distractions and worries.

9. Use Props: Consider using yoga props like blocks, straps, or bolsters to support your practice.

10. Listen to Your Body: Respect your body's limits and avoid pushing yourself into discomfort or pain.

11. Practice Regularly: Consistency is key. Try to practice somatic yoga regularly to experience its benefits.

12. Breathe Deeply: Deep, controlled breathing can help release tension and improve relaxation.

13. Explore Gentle Twists: Incorporate gentle twisting movements to release tension in the spine.

14. **Balance Asymmetry:** Pay attention to any imbalances in your body and work on restoring balance through your practice.

15. **Progress Gradually:** If you're new to somatic yoga, start with basic movements and progress to more advanced poses over time.

16. **Use Mirrors Sparingly:** While mirrors can be helpful for alignment, try to rely on your body's proprioception (awareness of body position) more.

17. **Focus on Sensation:** Rather than striving for perfect poses, focus on the sensations and feelings in your body.

18. **Practice Mindful Walking:** Incorporate mindful walking into your routine, paying attention to each step.

19. **Savasana is Essential:** Always include a final relaxation (Savasana) at the end of your practice to integrate your experiences.

20. Modify Poses: Don't hesitate to modify poses to suit your body's needs and limitations.

21. Explore Somatic Movements: Learn and explore specific somatic movements that target areas of tension.

22. Combine Somatics with Yoga: Integrate somatic movements into your regular yoga practice for added benefits.

23. Progressive Muscle Relaxation: Practice progressive muscle relaxation to release tension from head to toe.

24. Stay Hydrated: Drink water before and after your practice to stay hydrated.

25. Incorporate Mindfulness Meditation: Combine somatic yoga with mindfulness meditation for a holistic experience.

26. Seek Guidance: Consider taking classes or workshops with certified somatic yoga instructors.

27. Journal Your Experience: Keep a journal to document your progress, insights, and feelings during your practice.

28. Share with a Friend: Practice somatic yoga with a friend or partner to enhance your experience.

29. Practice Self-Compassion: Be gentle with yourself and avoid self-criticism during your practice.

30. Enjoy the Journey: Remember that somatic yoga is a journey of self-discovery and self-care. Enjoy the process and the benefits it brings to your body and mind.

30 DAY CHALLENGE SOMATIC YOGA EXERCISE

Day 1: Introduction to Breath Awareness

- Exercise: Begin with a 10-minute seated meditation focusing on your breath. Observe each inhale and exhale.

Day 2: Mindful Body Scan

- Exercise: Practice a 15-minute body scan meditation, paying attention to sensations in different body parts.

Day 3: Gentle Neck Rolls

- Exercise: Perform slow and gentle neck rolls, 5 rolls in each direction, to release neck tension.

Day 4: Cat-Cow Stretch

- Exercise: Incorporate 5 rounds of cat-cow stretches to warm up the spine.

Day 5: Seated Forward Bend

- Exercise: Practice a seated forward bend for 5 breath cycles to stretch the hamstrings and lower back.

Day 6: Child's Pose

- Exercise: Spend 10 minutes in child's pose, focusing on relaxation and deep breathing.

Day 7: Somatic Shoulder Rolls

- Exercise: Perform somatic shoulder rolls to release tension, 10 rolls in each direction.

Day 8: Mountain Pose with Breath Awareness

- Exercise: Stand in mountain pose and focus on breath awareness for 10 minutes.

Day 9: Somatic Hip Circles

- Exercise: Practice somatic hip circles to release hip tension, 10 circles in each direction.

Day 10: Tree Pose

- Exercise: Explore tree pose to improve balance and concentration, hold for 5 breath cycles on each leg.

Day 11: Somatic Spinal Twists

- Exercise: Perform somatic spinal twists to release tension, 10 twists on each side.

Day 12: Sphinx Pose

- Exercise: Spend 10 minutes in sphinx pose to gently stretch the lower back.

Day 13: Mindful Walking Meditation

- Exercise: Practice mindful walking meditation for 15 minutes, paying attention to each step.

Day 14: Seated Twist

- Exercise: Perform a seated twist on each side, holding for 5 breath cycles.

Day 15: Half Bridge Pose

- Exercise: Practice half bridge pose for 5 breath cycles to strengthen the lower back.

Day 16: Somatic Side Bends

- Exercise: Perform somatic side bends to release tension, 10 bends on each side.

Day 17: Warrior I Pose

- Exercise: Explore warrior I pose to improve strength and balance, hold for 5 breath cycles on each side.

Day 18: Somatic Pelvic Tilts

- Exercise: Practice somatic pelvic tilts to release tension, 10 tilts in each direction.

Day 19: Seated Meditation

- Exercise: Meditate in a seated position for 15 minutes, focusing on your breath.

Day 20: Downward Dog Pose

- Exercise: Practice downward dog pose for 5 breath cycles to stretch the entire body.

Day 21: Somatic Leg Circles

- Exercise: Perform somatic leg circles to release tension, 10 circles on each leg.

Day 22: Somatic Arm Waves

- Exercise: Practice somatic arm waves to release tension, 10 waves with each arm.

Day 23: Warrior II Pose

- Exercise: Explore warrior II pose to improve strength and balance, hold for 5 breath cycles on each side.

Day 24: Seated Forward Bend with Twist

- Exercise: Perform a seated forward bend with a twist on each side, holding for 5 breath cycles.

Day 25: Bridge Pose

- Exercise: Practice bridge pose for 5 breath cycles to strengthen the back and legs.

Day 26: Mindful Eating

- Exercise: Practice mindful eating during one meal, savoring each bite and paying attention to taste and texture.

Day 27: Somatic Knee Circles

- Exercise: Perform somatic knee circles to release tension, 10 circles in each direction.

Day 28: Extended Triangle Pose

- Exercise: Explore extended triangle pose to improve flexibility and strength, hold for 5 breath cycles on each side.

Day 29: Seated Meditation with Body Scan

- Exercise: Meditate in a seated position for 20 minutes, incorporating a body scan.

Day 30: Full Body Relaxation

- Exercise: Spend 20 minutes in savasana, focusing on full-body relaxation and deep breathing.

Day 31: Somatic Head-to-Toe Scan

- Exercise: Perform a somatic head-to-toe body scan, focusing on releasing tension throughout the body.

Day 32: Seated Twist and Forward Bend

- Exercise: Combine a seated twist and forward bend on each side, holding for 5 breath cycles.

Day 33: Somatic Arm Circles

- Exercise: Practice somatic arm circles to release tension, 10 circles with each arm.

Day 34: Warrior III Pose

- Exercise: Explore warrior III pose to improve balance and core strength, hold for 5 breath cycles on each leg.

Day 35: Seated Breath Awareness

- Exercise: Meditate in a seated position for 15 minutes, focusing solely on your breath.

Day 36: Somatic Spinal Waves

- Exercise: Perform somatic spinal waves to release tension, 10 waves of the spine.

Day 37: Somatic Hip Swings

- Exercise: Practice somatic hip swings to release hip tension, 10 swings on each side.

Day 38: Seated Side Stretch

- Exercise: Perform a seated side stretch on each side, holding for 5 breath cycles.

Day 39: Plank Pose

- Exercise: Practice plank pose for 5 breath cycles to strengthen the core.

Day 40: Mindful Body Scan and Breath Awareness

- Exercise: Combine a mindful body scan with breath awareness meditation for 20 minutes.

Day 41: Somatic Shoulder Shrugs

- Exercise: Perform somatic shoulder shrugs to release tension, 10 shrugs in each direction.

Day 42: Camel Pose

- Exercise: Explore camel pose to open the chest and improve flexibility, hold for 5 breath cycles.

Day 43: Seated Meditation with Loving-Kindness

- Exercise: Meditate in a seated position for 20 minutes, incorporating a loving-kindness meditation.

Day 44: Somatic Leg Swings

- Exercise: Practice somatic leg swings to release tension, 10 swings on each leg.

Day 45: Warrior I and Warrior II Flow

- Exercise: Flow between warrior I and warrior II poses for 10 breath cycles on each side.

Day 46: Seated Forward Bend with Twist and Stretch

- Exercise: Combine a seated forward bend with a twist and a stretch on each side, holding for 5 breath cycles.

Day 47: Dolphin Pose

- Exercise: Practice dolphin pose for 5 breath cycles to strengthen the shoulders and core.

Day 48: Mindful Walking in Nature

- Exercise: Take a mindful walk in nature for 30 minutes, connecting with the environment.

Day 49: Somatic Arm Twists

- Exercise:

 Perform somatic arm twists to release tension, 10 twists with each arm.

Day 50: Somatic Hip Circles and Squats

- Exercise: Combine somatic hip circles with squats for a lower body release, 10 circles in each direction and 10 squats.

Day 51: Warrior Flow and Balance

- Exercise: Flow between warrior I, warrior II, and warrior III poses for 10 breath cycles on each side.

Day 52: Seated Meditation with Body Scan and Breath Awareness

- Exercise: Meditate in a seated position for 30 minutes, incorporating a body scan and breath awareness.

Day 53: Somatic Shoulder and Neck Release

- Exercise: Perform somatic movements to release tension in the shoulders and neck, 10 repetitions.

Day 54: Pigeon Pose

- Exercise: Explore pigeon pose to release tension in the hips, hold for 5 breath cycles on each side.

Day 55: Seated Breath Awareness and Mindfulness

- Exercise: Meditate in a seated position for 20 minutes, combining breath awareness and mindfulness.

Day 56: Somatic Leg Swings and Hip Circles

- Exercise: Combine somatic leg swings and hip circles for a full lower body release, 10 swings and circles on each side.

Day 57: Sun Salutation

- Exercise: Practice a sun salutation sequence for 10 rounds to increase overall flexibility and strength.

Day 58: Seated Meditation with Gratitude

- Exercise: Meditate in a seated position for 20 minutes, incorporating a gratitude meditation.

Day 59: Somatic Full Body Integration

- Exercise: Perform a full-body somatic integration routine, focusing on releasing tension from head to toe.

Day 60: Reflect and Celebrate

- Exercise: Take time to reflect on your 60-day journey of somatic yoga. Celebrate your progress and set new intentions for your continued practice.

CONCLUSION

Embarking on a 60-day somatic yoga exercise challenge is a journey towards greater self-awareness, relaxation, and overall well-being. Throughout this challenge, you've explored a variety of somatic movements, yoga poses, and mindfulness practices, gradually deepening your connection with your body and breath.

Somatic yoga encourages you to be present in each moment, listen to your body's cues, and release tension gently. It's not about perfection but about self-care and self-discovery. By incorporating these practices into your daily routine, you've taken important steps toward a more balanced and mindful life.

As you conclude this 60-day challenge, remember that your somatic yoga journey doesn't have to end here. You can continue to explore and deepen your practice, integrating these techniques into your daily life to promote relaxation, reduce stress, and enhance your overall quality of life.

I would like to express my heartfelt gratitude for entrusting me with the opportunity to guide you through this 60-day somatic yoga exercise challenge. Your commitment to self-care and well-being is truly commendable.

It has been a pleasure to assist you on this journey, and I hope that you've found value in the exercises and practices you've explored. Remember that the benefits of somatic yoga extend beyond the physical; they touch the realms of mental and emotional well-being as well.

As you continue your path of self-discovery and mindful living, know that I am here to support you whenever you seek guidance or have questions. Your dedication to self-improvement is inspiring, and I'm excited to see where your continued somatic yoga practice takes you.

Thank you for choosing to prioritize your health and wellness. May your future endeavors be filled with peace, balance, and a deeper connection with yourself.

DR. PERSIS HILLARY

www.ingramcontent.com/pod-product-compliance
Lightning Source LLC
Chambersburg PA
CBHW061008260726

48661CB00005B/2104